SEVENTH EDITION

if your child stutters

a guide for parents

if your child stutters: a guide for parents

Publication No. 0011

Sixth Edition – 2002
Seventh Edition– 2006

Published by

Stuttering Foundation of America
3100 Walnut Grove, Suite 603
P. O. Box 11749
Memphis, Tennessee 38111-0749

ISBN 0-933388-58-9

The Stuttering Foundation of America is a nonprofit
charitable organization dedicated to the prevention
and treatment of stuttering.

To the Parent

This book is written for parents who are concerned about the speech of their young child. If your child usually speaks well but sometimes repeats words, sounds, or syllables, you may be afraid he or she is beginning to stutter. The goals of this book are to help you distinguish between normal disfluencies and stuttering and to enable you to begin working with your child with a better understanding of the problem.

1) **Educate yourself** about stuttering. The more you know, the more you can help your child and the less panicked you will feel.

2) **Start right away**. We now know that early intervention in preschool children is the key to keeping a minor problem from becoming a major one. Changes **you** make can make a difference.

3) **Find competent help**. If the problem persists, learn how to choose a therapist who is right for your child.

This book represents the thoughts of many experts in the field of stuttering, all of whom attach great importance to early intervention in prevention of stuttering in the young child.

Speech disorders can be frustrating as well as demoralizing, particularly when neglected or misunderstood. For this reason, every effort towards a deeper understanding of them will contribute significantly to your child's normal, healthy development and well-being.

Jane Fraser
President

Stuttering Foundation

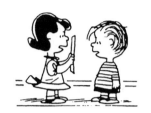

The Stuttering Foundation of America owes its thanks to Charles Schulz, creator of PEANUTS cartoons, for sharing Lucy and Linus with us. We feel that their presence has greatly enhanced this publication.

Professionals Who Contributed To This Book

Stanley Ainsworth, Ph.D., Author
> Distinguished Professor Emeritus of Speech Correction, University of Georgia.

Edward G. Conture, Ph.D.
> Professor, Department of Communication Sciences and Disorders, Vanderbilt University.

Carl Dell, Jr., Ph.D.
> Professor, Eastern Illinois University, Charleston, Illinois.

Jane Fraser, Co-author
> President, Stuttering Foundation of America.

Harold L. Luper, Ph.D.
> Formerly Professor and Head, Department of Audiology and Speech Pathology, University of Tennessee.

David Prins, Ph.D.
> Professor and Chairman, Department of Speech and Hearing Sciences, University of Washington, Seattle.

Harold B. Starbuck, Ph.D.
> Formerly Professor and Chairman, Department of Speech Pathology and Audiology, State University of New York, Geneseo, New York.

C. Woodruff Starkweather, Ph.D.
> Chairman Emeritus, Speech Sciences Division, Temple University, Philadelphia, Pennsylvania.

Lisa Scott, Ph.D.
> Assistant Professor, Florida State University.

Charles Van Riper, Ph.D.
> Distinguished Professor Emeritus, Western Michigan University.

Dean E. Williams, Ph.D.
> Professor Emeritus, University of Iowa.

Table of Contents

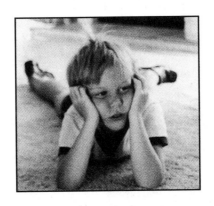

Part **I**

does my child stutter?

Speech begins with the first cry at birth. It then develops rapidly during the first two years as the child learns to make meaningful sounds and words. Later, between the ages of 2 and 6, he may begin to have noticeable difficulties in speaking smoothly and freely, especially when starting to use sentences. All children repeat words and phrases, hesitate often, and have occasional difficulty with the smooth flow of words, but some have more trouble than others and for longer periods of time.

> All children repeat, hesitate, and have occasional difficulty with the smooth flow of words, but some have more trouble than others and for longer periods of time.

If your child has been having this type of trouble, you may wonder if he or she is beginning to stutter. Will it get worse or will it go away? If you think your child is stuttering, should you do something, and if so, what?

Our aim is to answer some of these questions.

Is It Stuttering?

Stuttering interrupts the flow of speech, but so do many other things. All of us repeat words or syllables occasionally; no one has speech that is perfectly smooth. We all hesitate, insert noises or words, get syllables mixed up, go back and revise sentences, or try to say two words at the same time. When these things happen, we end up confused or stuck for an instant.

The young child who is just learning to talk will naturally stumble more often than adults and older children. The smoothness or fluency of everyone's speech also varies tremendously with internal feelings and external circumstances. These variations in fluency are more extreme in the young child.

Because children with normal disfluencies show many of the same behaviors found in stuttering, it may be difficult for you to distinguish them from stuttering. Moreover, these vary in severity and frequency depending on time, circumstance, and the feelings of the speaker.

Therefore, if you are concerned about your child's speech, it is probably best to let a speech-language pathologist determine whether your child is actually stuttering. Regardless, whether he is or not, the suggestions in this book should be helpful to you.

How to Decide if Your Child is Beginning to Stutter

Certain signs indicate a child is in the beginning stages of stuttering. Understanding these signs will help you decide whether a visit to a speech-language pathologist is necessary.

After reading this book, you may decide to take your child to see a speech-language pathologist.* During a speech evaluation, some children do not display some or even any of the things that have concerned their parents. Therefore, if you decide to see a therapist, your knowledge of the signs of early stuttering together with your day-to-day contact with your child make you the best source of information. You can describe how your child talks, as

---

*The Stuttering Foundation at 1-800-992-9392 and www.stutteringhelp.org (www.tartamudez.org in Spanish) will provide you with the names of speech-language pathologists who specialize in stuttering. In addition, agencies that may provide speech testing and therapy include your local school district (contact your local elementary school for more information), a hospital clinic (look under "Outpatient Services" or "Speech Therapy"), or a speech and hearing clinic at a nearby university.

No matter whom you choose, be sure to ask:
- Have you / has the therapist who will see my child had a lot of experience working with those who stutter?
- Are you / is this therapist experienced in working with children?
- Do you / does the therapist have certification from the American Speech-Language-Hearing Association (CCC-SLP)?

well as how often and how consistently the disfluencies occur. This information is important in helping the speech pathologist determine whether your child is stuttering. Remember, when it comes to your own child, *you* are the expert.

Warning Signs*

Stuttering is more than just disruptions in the smooth flow of words, which we refer to as *disfluencies*. It is also reactions to difficulty speaking. There are a few key warning signs to look for when trying to decide whether your child might be stuttering. When you consider these warning signs, try to avoid becoming too conscious of them. See them in relation to your child's total speech, most of which is probably quite fluent.

Also, keep in mind that many of these behaviors come and go. They occur at times in children who are never thought of as stutterers.

1. Multiple Repetitions

Keep in mind that many of these behaviors come and go.

All of us, particularly children learning to talk, repeat words and phrases. It is not uncommon for a 3 year old to repeat one word several times.

"Is-is-is it time to go yet?"

One child, who was not a stutterer, repeated "and-and-and-and-and..." so many times that he forgot what he wanted to say. Fortunately, he laughed about it and so did his parents.

Sometimes, "starter" words or sounds such as a prolonged or repeated "er" or "um" are used.

"Um, um, um, can I have one of the cookies?"

Also, parts of words, usually the first syllable, may be repeated.

"Can I have my ba-ba-ba-baby?"

---

*These warning signs are presented in a DVD entitled *Stuttering and Your Child: Help for Parents,* produced by The Stuttering Foundation. This 30-minute DVD may be purchased from The Stuttering Foundation, P.O. Box 11749, Memphis, TN 38111-0749 or viewed free online at www.stutteringhelp.org.

If your child begins to frequently use these repetitions with many words and in many situations, he or she may be having more difficulty than normal with his speech. The use of these repetitions may be a passing phase. It is, however, one of the first signs a clinician looks for when deciding whether your child may be stuttering.

2. Schwa Vowel

The schwa (or weak) vowel is used in many everyday words. It is the "uh" sound heard in unstressed syllables such as "around," "concerned," "suggest," "wanted," and "the boy."

The child who is beginning to stutter often uses the schwa in a way that distorts the word. If he says "go-go-go-goat," we don't worry. But if he says

"guh-guh-guh-goat,"

we identify this as a warning sign, particularly if he repeats the schwa sound very quickly. In words that begin with a vowel, such as "over," he may say

"uh-uh-uh-over,"

instead of repeating the initial sound "o." You may have difficulty in distinguishing these differences, but the therapist is trained to do so.

3. Prolongations

Sometimes, instead of repeating initial sounds, your child may prolong the first sound of a word, so that "Mommy" becomes

"Mmmmmmmmmmmmommy."

These first three signs—repeating sounds, repeating the schwa, and prolonging sounds—may occur occasionally in nearly all children. If they begin to occur too frequently in too many speaking situations and begin to affect your child's ability to communicate, you should be concerned.

4. Tremors

Occasionally you may notice that the small muscles around your child's mouth and jaw tremble or vibrate when she seems to get stuck on words. The degree of tremor may be mild or intense. These tremors are associated with difficulties in moving forward with speech when her mouth is held in one position with no sound coming out. The therapist will want to know how often you have noticed these tremors and if they appear to be lasting longer now than before.

5. Rise in Pitch and Loudness

As your child tries to get a word out, his pitch and loudness may rise before he finishes the word. It may slide upwards or suddenly jump to a higher level. In both cases, he is trying to get the stuck word unstuck, but again this is a sign that he needs help.

6. Struggle and Tension

Your child may struggle to get words out or have an unusual amount of tension in his lips, tongue, throat or chest when she tries to say certain words. At other times she may have only a small amount of necessary tension on the very same words. The degree of struggle may vary from being hardly noticeable to very obvious in certain speaking situations, and may disappear entirely for long periods of time. In any event, struggle and tension indicate your child is having greater difficulty with speaking.

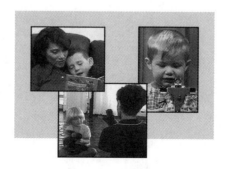

7. Moment of Fear

You may see a fleeting moment of fear or frustration in your child's face as he approaches a word. If so, he has probably experienced enough difficulty getting stuck to make him react emotionally to the anticipation of trouble. He may go beyond momentary fear and begin to cry because he can't say a word. If you can help your child while the fear is still a brief passing experience, there is a good chance of preventing a vivid or lasting fear of speaking from developing.

8. Avoidance

Struggling to speak and being afraid to talk may lead your child to avoid talking. She may postpone trying to say a word until she is sure she can say it fluently. She may refuse to talk at times, substituting or inserting words or that are not really part of the sentence. She will continue to have normal delays in speaking as she tries to choose words or formulate sentences but the delays may take longer. If she does not speak even when it is clear that she knows what she wants to say, she is probably avoiding because of her growing frustration with talking.

You may observe these last five behaviors—tremors, rise in pitch and loudness, struggle and tension, moment of fear, and avoidance—in your child. They occur when he or she begins to react to interruptions in speech, and usually mean that your child is trying to do something about the interruptions. Again, if you observe these behaviors, you should be concerned.

14

Risk Factors

Some factors place a child at risk for stuttering. Knowing these factors will help you try to decide whether or not your child needs to see a speech-language pathologist[1,2].

1. Family History

There is now strong evidence that almost half of all children who stutter have a family member who stutters. The risk that your child is actually stuttering instead of just having normal disfluencies increases if that family member is still stuttering. There is less risk if the family member outgrew stuttering as a child.

2. Age at onset

Children who begin stuttering before age $3\frac{1}{2}$ are more likely to outgrow stuttering; if your child begins stuttering before age 3, there is a much better chance she will outgrow it within 6 months.

3. Time since onset

Between 75% and 80% of all children who begin stuttering will stop within 12 to 24 months without speech therapy. If your child has been stuttering longer than 6 months, he may be less likely to outgrow it on his own. If he has been stuttering longer than 12 months, there is an even smaller likelihood he will outgrow it on his own.

---

[1]Longitudinal research studies by Drs. Ehud Yairi and Nicoline G. Ambrose and colleagues at the University of Illinois provide excellent new information about the development of stuttering in early childhood. Their findings are helping speech-language pathologists determine who is most likely to outgrow stuttering versus who is most likely to develop a lifelong stuttering problem. Research reports include:

Yairi, E. & Ambrose, N. (1992). A longitudinal study of stuttering in children: A preliminary report. *Journal of Speech, Language, and Hearing Research, 35,* 755-760.

Ambrose, N. & Yairi, E. (1999). Normative disfluency data for early childhood stuttering. *Journal of Speech, Language, and Hearing Research, 42,* 895-909.

Yairi, E. & Ambrose, N. (1999). Early childhood stuttering I: Persistence and recovery rates. *Journal of Speech, Language, and Hearing Research, 42,* 1097-1112.

[2]Yairi, E. & Ambrose, N. (2005). *Early Childhood Stuttering: For Clinicians by Clinicians,* ProEd, Austin, TX.

4. Gender

Girls are more likely than boys to outgrow stuttering. In fact, three to four boys continue to stutter for every girl who stutters.

Why this difference? First, it appears that during early childhood, there are innate differences between boys' and girls' speech and language abilities. Second, during this same period, parents, family members, and others often react to boys somewhat differently than girls. Therefore, it may be that more boys stutter than girls because of basic differences in boys' speech and language abilities *and* differences in their interactions with others.

That being said, many boys who begin stuttering will outgrow the problem. What is important for you to remember is that if your child is stuttering right now, it doesn't necessarily mean he or she will stutter the rest of his or her life.

5. Other speech and language factors

A child who speaks clearly with few, if any, speech errors would be more likely to outgrow stuttering than a child whose speech errors make him difficult to understand. If your child makes frequent speech errors such as substituting one sound for another or leaving sounds out of words, or has trouble following directions, you should be more concerned.

The most recent findings dispel previous reports that children who begin stuttering have, as a group, lower language skills. On the contrary, there are indications that they are well within the norms or above. Advanced language skills appear to be even more of a risk factor for children whose stuttering persists.[1]

---

[1]Yairi, E. & Ambrose, N. (2005). *Early Childhood Stuttering: For Clinicians by Clinicians,* Chapter 7, Pro-Ed, Austin, TX.

Risk Factor Chart

Place a check next to each that is true for your child

Risk Factor	More likely in beginning stuttering	True for My Child
Family history of stuttering	A parent, sibling, or other family member who still stutters	
Age at onset	After age 3½	
Time since onset	Stuttering 6–12 months or longer	
Gender	Male	
Other speech-language concerns	Speech sound errors, trouble being understood, difficulty following directions	

These risk factors place children at higher risk for stuttering. If your child has any of these risk factors and is showing some or all of the warning signs mentioned previously, you should be more concerned. You may want to schedule a speech screening with a speech therapist who specializes in stuttering. The therapist will decide whether your child is stuttering, and then determine whether to wait a bit longer or begin treatment right away.

Sometimes the speech-language pathologist will suggest that you listen for particular things. Try to listen objectively. This may be difficult, but it can be learned. If you are going to observe your child's speech more closely over a period of time, there are certain things you should be aware of:

- As in other areas of development, speech does not progress evenly. You will probably notice more difficulty at some times than at others. Some children stutter more when tired, sick, or out of their normal daily routine.

- Pay special attention to periods of more fluent speech. This will help you be less anxious about the occasional difficulty. Many children are much more fluent than disfluent, but it's easy to pay too much attention to the behavior that has you worried.

- Don't try to observe her every time she opens her mouth. Pay attention to *what* she is trying to tell you rather than *how* she is saying it. It's important for your child to know you are interested and understand her when she talks.

- Try to judge the amount of difficulty he is having and whether the speech is getting better or worse on the whole.

- Some parents find it helpful to make a daily rating on their calendar. For example, one mother used a scale of 1 to 7 with 1 being a very fluent day, 7 being a day with lots of stuttering. Every day, she would rate her child's fluency and put the rating on her calendar. Over time, she saw that the ratings were improving and felt less worried about her son. These ratings will also be helpful to the speech-language pathologist.

The Speech Evaluation

The speech evaluation is used to determine whether or not your child needs treatment for stuttering. The speech-language pathologist will use information from several sources to determine whether your child is at risk for stuttering and the best course of action to take.

First, the therapist will probably ask you to fill out a case history. This form may cover:

- Developmental milestones;
- Medical history;
- Speech development;
- Family history of stuttering, if any;
- Information about past therapy, if any;
- Your impressions of your child and his or her speech;
- Family interaction styles and schedules;
- Other concerns you may have regarding your child's development.

This is usually followed by a family interview during which the therapist will ask you about your child's speech development, your concerns, and family routines. The therapist may also ask you about your child's reactions to different situations and his basic temperament. This is also a time for you to ask questions.

During the actual assessment, your child may be videotaped talking to you, the therapist or other staff. The therapist may also have asked you to bring in a video or audio sample of your child talking at home, if possible. The therapist will use these tapes to carefully observe your child's speech. Other aspects of your child's speech, such as grammar, vocabulary, and speech sounds, will also be examined.

In short, as much information as possible about your child will be collected before a recommendation is made regarding the need for treatment.

After the assessment, the therapist will likely schedule a follow-up appointment to discuss his or her findings and whether speech therapy is needed, or whether it would be best to wait and further monitor your child's speech. Be sure to use this important time to share your concerns and ask questions.

Finally, the therapist will provide a written report of the evaluation and recommendations. This may be used by your pediatrician or by your insurance company if a referral is required for insurance reimbursement. See page 60 for more information on insurance reimbursement.

Within the field of speech pathology, honest opinions may differ on when, or whether, to start therapy. As a parent, you know your child best. If you receive "wait and see" advice from a speech-language pathologist or a pediatrician, but are still concerned, be persistent and follow your instincts.

Continue to pay attention to your child's speech. Seek another opinion. If your pediatrician is looking for more information, *The Child Who Stutters: To the Pediatrician,* is available free online from The Stuttering Foundation.* It is an excellent source of information to help your doctor make the right referral decision for your child.

Meanwhile, the advice in this book gives you excellent ways to **begin helping your child today.**

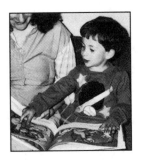

*www.stutteringhelp.org and www.tartamudez.org

Part **II**

what causes stuttering?

This is a frustrating question because in spite of the many things we know about stuttering, we cannot provide a clear-cut answer. It seems that children stutter for many reasons which vary from one child to the next and that stuttering sometimes continues when early causes are no longer in effect.

> Children stutter for many reasons. These reasons vary from one child to the next and stuttering sometimes continues even after early causes are no longer in effect.

The Role of Inheritance

As described in Part I, stuttering seems to run in some families. Does this mean that stuttering is inherited? Scientists have found what seems to be a genetic base for stuttering in about half of all children who stutter. The role of inheritance is quite complex, however, and not as predictable as the inheritance of eye or hair color.

Muscle Coordination

Evidence also shows that some children have basic problems managing the fine coordination and timing sequences of the movements needed for fluent speech, especially during the early years as their neuromuscular system develops.

[1] Yairi, et al, 1996, Drayna 1997

Lack of coordination in speech may cause disfluency, just as poor coordination of large muscles may cause tripping or falling while the child is learning to walk. Stuttering may continue as the child learns to control speech muscles, although in some children it may fade away. This leads us to believe that other factors must account for the continued development of stuttering.

Environmental-Emotional Stress

Certain kinds of emotional stress—either a single very upsetting event or a continuing pattern of stress—can disrupt speech patterns in most of us. The young child is particularly vulnerable because he is still learning to manage his emotions and many things seem threatening to him. Some children are particularly sensitive to changes in their emotions or environment and get upset more easily. The child may begin to fear certain speaking situations because in his mind they are similar to others that were difficult. Not all children who undergo similar experiences begin to stutter, however.

Some children even react negatively to normal disfluencies. These negative reactions from the child herself or those around her may make her feel like disfluencies are bad and she should stop them from happening. The more she tries to stop, the worse they become, which may lead to more negative reactions. A vicious cycle may begin that leads to increased stress, worry, and tension when she starts to say something.

You may have wondered if your child could be stuttering because of an intensely frightening experience. Although this could be the reason for some initial disruption in speech, it usually has only a temporary effect.

Imitation

Can stuttering be "caught" through imitation? Based on current understanding of speech and related events, imitation is an overly simplistic explanation for the cause of an extremely complex problem.

Now you see why we cannot say for sure, "This is why young children stutter," but we do know many of the things that make it develop into a serious problem. Some concern your child; but others involve you.

You have not caused your child to stutter, but certainly there are steps you can take to keep it from developing into a more serious problem.

Stuttering cannot be "caught" through imitation.

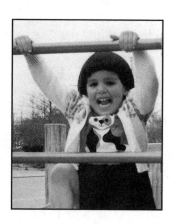

Part III

additional facts about stuttering

How Many People Stutter?

Stutterers account for about one percent of the population, but a higher percentage of young children go through a temporary period of stuttering. Although one percent seems rather small, it does mean that approximately three million people in the United States stutter.

How Does the Child Who Stutters Compare With Those Who Do Not?

Aside from their stuttering, most children who stutter are quite normal. They range in intelligence just as the rest of us do.

Researchers have tried to find physical and psychological differences between those who stutter and those who don't. The few differences that have been found are very subtle, are contradicted by other studies, and do not appear consistently in all those who stutter.

The young child, at least, seems to be as well adjusted as his non-stuttering friends. You may notice that your child is especially sensitive, gets upset or frustrated easily, or is more active than other children but these things may or may not be related to the way he speaks.

Recovery from Stuttering

Many very young children stop stuttering without any treatment or special attention at all. It has been estimated that for every person who stutters today, there are three to four people who have stuttered at some point in their development. In Part I of this book, we used a chart to help you decide whether your child might be at risk for stuttering. Here are the things we know about recovery in young children:

- Children with a family history of stuttering are less likely to recover.

- Sometimes recovery can take as long as three years after stuttering is first noticed. However, most children will recover from stuttering within one year.

- Children who begin stuttering after age 3 1/2 are less likely to recover.

- Boys are less likely to recover than girls.

- Children with other speech/language concerns are less likely to recover.

Other factors also influence how quickly recovery takes place. Stress and anxiety almost always aggravate stuttering in a young child.

For this reason, many suggestions for helping your child are aimed at reducing these as much as possible. The hard part is finding out your child's source of anxiety or stress. Many children, once they are under less stress or feel less anxiety, will be more fluent. But if your child has been stuttering for more than three to six months, professional help may be needed.

Stuttering Swings Like a Pendulum

We know that the frequency and severity of stuttering usually varies with time and circumstance. Sometimes your child will talk easily, such as when he is speaking to himself, to pets, or while singing. The stuttering may disappear completely for relatively long periods of time and then return in full force. This may happen when stress and anxiety increase, but not always. If your child's stuttering continues to come and go like this over a longer period of time, you should be more concerned.

Some "Good" Advice is Bad

We also know that many of the old traditional methods of reacting to stuttering do not help. In fact, they may make the problem worse. Telling your child to "Talk slowly," to "Take a deep breath," or to "Relax," are some examples of useless suggestions. Instructions to "Say it again," may result in your child saying it fluently but this will not make stuttering stop.

Even more harmful are loud orders such as "Stop that!" combined with harsh looks and punishment. These methods are based on one or more false assumptions about the nature of stuttering: that it is simply a bad habit which your child can stop if he really tries. Children do not stutter on purpose to be naughty or irritating.

- Do not say "slow down," but do learn to slow your **own** speech.

- Do not finish your child's sentences, but do allow your child to finish his or her own thoughts.

- Do not tell your child to "relax" or "say it again." Such simplistic advice isn't helpful, and may aggravate the problem if misused.

The next chapter explains in depth how to help your child.

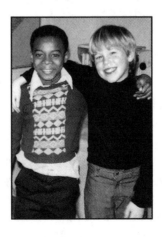

26

six ways to help your child

The interaction between you and your child is unique. In this section, we will offer you some helpful suggestions that may slightly change the way you interact with your child. Some are explicit instructions; others are more general and leave the details to you. Remember that the way you do something is as important as what you do. A simple list of "dos" and "don'ts" won't be effective unless it is based on what you believe. Also keep in mind that sometimes doing nothing may be the most important thing you can do.

Our suggestions directly relate to your child's ability to speak fluently and to

> The way you do something is as important as what you do.

interact freely with others. If you are concerned about your child's speech, the following suggestions are particularly important, but they also encourage the social development of any child.

All of the topics discussed involve direct changes in your own behavior and attitudes. This does not imply that if your child begins to stutter, it is your fault. We now know that parents do not cause stuttering, but once stuttering begins, there are many things that you can do to prevent it from becoming a lifelong problem. The one thing you can control and change is the most important part of your child's environment: you. For many very young children, certain changes made by you and other members of the family are the most effective way to encourage normal fluency.

A Note About Speech Development In General

Let's briefly review what to expect for speech development between the ages of two and six. This period represents an explosion of growth and development.

By the age of two, your child may be using words and short sentences consistently. By the age of six, he will be using longer sentences and a greater variety of words. He will also have begun to learn how to use his voice and words to control the behavior of others and to express his feelings. He will be using speech extensively in his social interactions.

Many new doors are opening rapidly and speech plays a central role in all of these. Your child needs to be understood, and needs to be able to say what she wants, when she wants to.

Suggestion 1: Listen with "All Ears"

It may surprise you that changing how you listen is one of the most important things you can do to help your child. Of course you listen to your child; it's hard not to as he is chattering or questioning you constantly. You may already listen selectively, not always paying attention to everything your child says.

We can help you selectively listen in ways that do not give your child the impression that you never listen or don't want to listen to him. Furthermore, you can learn to become more aware of what is important to your child and his development.

Paying attention to listening itself as well as to your personal listening habits will lead to better communication with your child. There are four key steps to improve your listening. Use these steps over several days.

Step 1. Study How You Listen and React to Your Child

For the first two or three days, concentrate from time to time on evaluating just how you listen to him, how much, and how often. Note the different ways you listen: from hearing only a small part of what he is saying to giving full attention to almost every word.

- What kind of topics get your attention?
- Do you let him finish before you start talking?
- Do you hurry her when she tries to talk?
- How much of his chatter do you actually hear?
- How much does she talk and what does she talk to you about?
- How do you react when he interrupts you?
- How often do you look at her when you are actively listening?

Jot down some notes about how you listen. This attention to the way in which you listen will provide the basis for the next three steps.

Step 2. Begin to Change the Ways you Listen and React to Your Child

For the next day or two, try to change the balance of your listening. You cannot listen attentively every time he opens his mouth, nor should you, particularly if he talks a great deal; but you may decide that more or less attention is better in different situations. You may decide to change how much you listen in situations in which you did not listen attentively before.

If necessary, change the way you react when he interrupts you. Instead of ignoring him or getting upset, let him know you heard him but it's not his turn to talk right now, or that you are busy but can listen later. The important thing is to learn that you can change your listening habits.

Step 3. Try to Understand the Feelings Behind the Words

For the next few days, listen to the way your child is speaking. How does he use his voice to tell you how he's feeling or what he really means? Note his inflections on words, when he pauses, whether he repeats phrases or sentences to get your attention, the timing of words, and the way he looks or doesn't look at you.

- Does she talk in a whining tone with you and others?
- Does he sound fearful with some members of the family?
- Do you frequently hear an upward inflection in "Mommy" when she wants attention?
- Does he repeat words more often with some people than with others?
- When she talks to dolls, toys or imaginary playmates, does she use "bossy" tones that are different from the way she speaks to people?
- Does he frequently talk about certain topics or ask certain questions because of fears he may have?

These guidelines should help you listen in a more understanding way and react more appropriately to both literal word meanings and the important feelings behind them. This is the essence of being a good listener, a good communicator.

As you become more aware of when to listen carefully and when to pay less attention, you will find ways to let your child know that your varying attention to daily duties does not mean that you don't love him. Deliberately interrupt your other activities at times in order to express your love and interest. He'll learn that when he really needs your attention, you're willing and able to give it.

Step 4. Identify Situations Requiring Immediate Intense Listening

As a final step, try to identify any signal that your child sends indicating an immediate need for intensive listening. Vocal signals can be a drastic change in loudness or unusual hesitations and repetitions, and usually occur long before the noisy crying stage. These may take a long time to recognize because these occasions do not occur often. When they do occur, be alert to facial expressions, postures, and movements.

Because listening is such an important part of the communication process and because it is directly related to emotion, improving your listening habits should have a direct effect on your child's fluency. Remember that listening should be a rewarding and joyful experience—not a burden.

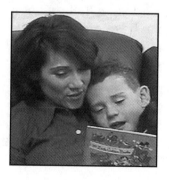

Suggestion 2: Talk *With* Rather Than *At* Your Child

How you talk and how you listen are closely related. At times, it seems you are continuously talking to your child: you must give information, set rules, discipline him, and otherwise manage his behavior with your voice and words. Even though you are constantly talking to him, in spite of yourself, you may find that you are talking at him most of the time. Instead of having a conversation where you each take turns sharing ideas and feelings, you do most of the talking.

It is not surprising that some children are more sensitive to this than others. You can help prevent an adverse reaction by making conscious efforts to counteract the amount of talking **at** with an increase in the periods of talking **with,** during which you are having a conversation with your child, exchanging ideas and feelings. Balanced in this way, talking becomes a sharing experience that is pleasant for both of you.

Talk About Things That Are Important to Your Child

Help your child by making talking an enjoyable experience.

First, listen to or tape record yourself during daily five-minute conversations for several days to determine how much time you spend talking **at** your child Then deliberately set up more time and topics for talking **with** her.

Talk with her about things that do not involve her behavior. Talking about what she has done during the day at preschool or daycare, about her favorite toys or about a book you are reading together are all good topics of conversation.

Let her know that you can and will listen patiently, and let her lead the talking as much as possible but never force it if she's having difficulty. Contribute to the conversation by commenting on the things your child is talking about; she will enjoy your attention and learn that talking can be fun.

Be a Good Speech Model for Your Child.

We assume that you are trying to provide examples of good speech for your child, that you speak clearly and use appropriate words for objects and events. We hope you use sentences and vocabulary appropriate for his age. Do you usually talk rapidly and fluently? If so, your child may be attempting to imitate you although he does not yet have the skills to do so, and thus naturally stumbles and hesitates.

If you think this is the case, make an effort to talk more slowly. Pause more often. If your sentences tend to be long, complex, or rambling, your child will probably have trouble understanding you and not know how to respond. This may lead to disfluencies when he replies. Try simpler and shorter sentences, at least part of the time.

Do you tend to interrupt him or cut off the ends of his sentences because you know what he is going to say? This adds unnecessary time pressure. Give him time: you can learn to act and speak with more patience. Tell him that Mom and Dad have time to listen.

Make Talking Fun.

You have already begun to make talking fun for your child when you listen in the way we have described, but you can do more. Singing while holding or rocking her is pleasant for both of you. Talk with her more about what you are doing while you are doing it, such as making dinner or folding laundry.

The more verbal fun you can have in the family, the more quickly your child will learn that speaking can be a pleasure. This should help offset the many times that speech must be used to scold, reprimand, or punish.

At certain times, be sure that the family pays attention to what he is saying. After all, brothers and sisters also need to learn to let others talk instead of always seizing attention. If your child begins to monopolize the conversation, she too may need to learn to let others speak. The important point is to avoid too many frustrating experiences.

Read or Tell Stories to Him.

Reading aloud and story telling also emphasize the pleasurable side of talking. They are important enough for some special attention.

Try to make a habit of reading aloud to your child on a regular basis, even if it's only for a few minutes each day. When you have read the same favorite stories many times, let him finish some of the sentences or tell the story to you in his own words, but only if he wants to.

If you feel you do not have a knack for making up stories, begin with favorite pictures, preferably those with a story behind them. Tell him about events from your own life when you were little or when he was smaller. All children love this.

Try to find an opportunity every day for "reading" pictures, reading books, or telling stories at a time when there are few or no interruptions. You can tell a silly story about something your child did when he was "little" while you're riding together in the car, or read a story to him while he's in the tub or while you're waiting for dinner to finish cooking. If you find yourself competing with the television, have a fixed time to turn it off. Even turning the TV off ten minutes a day to make time for reading or story telling can make a big difference.

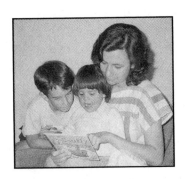

Help Her Express Her Feelings Verbally.

How often do you tell and show your child that you love or like her? It will be difficult for her to learn to express these very important feelings if you do not set the example.

What do you laugh at? If you tend to laugh at things that hurt others, you are teaching her to do the same. She needs to learn that there are several kinds of laughter, so talk with her about what made you laugh. Laugh at funny things, not hurtful things.

The next time she is angry, take the necessary time to listen to her. Talk about what it was that made her angry. There may be many reasons she's upset: being frustrated, demanding her own way, hurt feelings, or perhaps an imitation of your own displays of anger or fatigue.

Talk with her about better ways to express her feelings. Show her that she can get what she really wants without displays of temper, and teach her how to use words in a polite way. When she has found better ways of expressing her feelings, the conflicts causing some of her disfluencies will be reduced.

Eliminate "Command Performances."

Your efforts to force your child to talk can disrupt his fluency. You may want him to tell you what has happened in a situation or merely to tell Aunt Martha something interesting. It's also natural

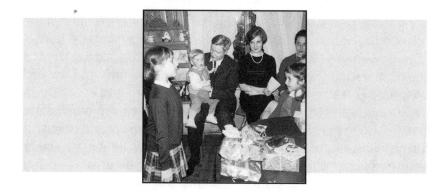

to demand that he say "please," and "thank you." Sometimes these "command performances" can produce disfluency because you are putting a great deal of pressure on him withoutrealizing it.

This extra pressure can be avoided by letting him proceed at his own rate. Instead of demanding that he say "please" and "thank you," make sure you model it by saying something like, "When someone gives us something, we say 'thank you,'" or, "It's nice manners to say 'please.'" As for talking about situations or telling Aunt Martha something interesting, is it really so important that she tell Aunt Martha at all?

Suggestion 3: Pay Attention to Body Language

Words are not the only way we communicate with others. A fundamental sense of well-being, or lack of it, is often communicated without words.

Most people think of communication as talking—words expressing thoughts or ideas. But it is far more. Perhaps you already know this but tend to forget its importance as your child grows older. Even before your child began to talk, he jabbered in a pattern that sounded like speech but with no understandable words. Nevertheless, he was communicating with you. If you responded to this, you both undoubtedly felt deep satisfaction.

As your child grows older, he continues to use first nonsense then recognizable words for this same emotional communication. Adults do the same; real words actually become non-words. We say "G'morning" without any thought to the meaning of each word. This is our way of reaching out to others.

If you listen carefully, you realize that your child often uses speech to reach out and make contact: "Mommy, my eye hurts!" "Daddy, see this big scratch on my leg?" Your specific answers to these questions are not as important as noticing and paying attention. Does he ask the same questions over and over? Does he always seem to want your attention while you are particularly busy? Asking the same questions or asking questions to which he already knows the answer are often signs that he simply wants your emotional attention. As you become more sensitive to the emotions that underlie so much of this kind of speech, you can respond in a more meaningful and appropriate way.

Seek Ways to Express Feelings Other Than by Talking.

Look at her and smile whenever you can. If she asks why you are smiling, tell her it is because you love her. Occasionally touch or pat her as she goes by you; the look on your face as well as your words will express your pride in her. Help her to do difficult things cheerfully but try not to demand verbal thanks from her.

Analyze How Your Child Uses His Voice.

Listen to his and to your own inflections, loudness, and pitch levels when you talk with him to see what they tell you about the emotions underlying speech. One way to do this is by turning on a tape recorder and letting it run until you have forgotten it is there; then listen to parts of the tape.

What are you listening for? Perhaps you already know how much louder you speak when you are angry with your child or stressed in general. You may find that you speak in a higher pitched voice, which at times becomes very harsh and grating. You may even notice unusual pitch patterns—upward and downward inflections—as you try to be patient but struggle to control your irritation. At times, you may hear a condescending tone, or talking down to your child.

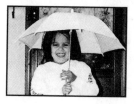 Perhaps your voice patterns are not extreme, but are they always the same when you speak to your child and usually different when you talk to others? Do you use a similar tone in speaking to your dog and to your child? Try to make modifications in your own speech in a way that emphasizes positive, constructive feelings.

Provide Time for Closeness.

You have no doubt treasured those moments when you have felt especially close to your child and when words between you were few—taking a walk, baking cookies, making dinner, fixing something, activities that demand little or no speech. If these moments occur often, even if they are brief, they will help her to feel more secure and stuttering may decrease.

These quiet happy times often occur accidentally, but you can create more of them. It may involve no more than sharing her play with blocks, picking up toys with her for a few moments, or walking together through the park.

Not everything you plan will produce the level of closeness you want, but you can gradually build a relationship that makes her aware of being wanted and loved without a constant flow of words. Words of love without the nonverbal demonstration of it are meaningless and a child soon learns this.

Suggestion 4: Make Day-to-Day Living Easier

There is more to bringing up your child than talking with him. Children have a variety of opportunities to grow more strong and secure or to feel more threatened and weak. We will not try to provide you with a comprehensive manual on all the problems of parenthood, but certain aspects of it contain many possibilities for promoting fluency.

Make Meal Time Less Stressful.

Minor changes in day-to-day activities can help promote fluency.

If your child is a fussy eater and mealtime is a problem for both of you, you may want to re-examine the situation.

- Does he stutter more at mealtime?
- What conflicts occur?
- Are you talking at him?
- Are you scolding frequently?
- Are you worried that he is not getting enough of the right foods?
- Are you too concerned about how he eats?
- Are you confusing eating and drinking with discipline?
- Are you using mealtime to discuss adult problems, such as work or money?

If he is provided with good food, is not nagged to eat it, and doesn't snack just before meals, he will eventually get hungry enough to eat what he needs. If he tends to lose his appetite at the usual time and place for meals, try changing things around for awhile. If you are working on manners, do it as a game while he is eating a dish of ice cream. The rest of the time, control your impulse to correct him. If you are using mealtime to discuss your adult problems, this should be done at a different time because he will be very sensitive to your own stress.

When mealtime becomes a struggle, he will always win—because you cannot make him eat. Don't try; all you will do is to make everyone miserable. You can control where and when he eats, and that is enough.

Establish a Bed Time Routine.

You can't make your child go to sleep either, and if you try, you may find that she is in control of the going-to-bed process. Many children will stall getting in to bed by using delaying tactics: asking for a drink of water, begging you to read one more page in the book, having you check for scary monsters under the bed after you've already done so many times. We are sure you are familiar with many of the delaying tactics your child uses.

The key to reducing struggles at bedtime lies in being consistent. Make getting ready for bed as simple as possible. Evening is often a good time to read to her, but this can be done earlier rather than at the last minute. Hold her in your arms as a way of calming her just before she goes to bed. Make rules about how many drinks are allowed, how many pages will be read, or how many times you will come into her room after you've put her down, and stick to the rules. Be as consistent as possible.

Monitor Toilet Training.

Toilet training can be a difficult process. Since you can't *make* your child go to the toilet or control all the accidents, don't try. If you're not sure when to begin toilet training, ask your doctor about the best time to start. Some children toilet train quickly; others take much longer.

The important thing is that you treat your child in such a way that he is not made to feel he is a failure if he has an accident or wets the bed. You can help him see that in spite of the mess it creates, accidents are OK and that learning to use the toilet is just a part of growing up. By reducing his feelings of guilt, you make it easier for him and for yourself in the long run.

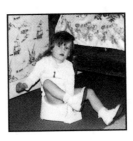

Reduce Pressure.

Examine the daily activities in which your family is involved.

- Is there so much going on that your child is bounced from one thing to another simply because the rest of the family is so involved in them?

- If she goes to preschool, what is her schedule there?

- How can you balance it at home so that she gets necessary rest and activity?

- Does she have periodic quiet times at school and at home, or does she have so much time to herself that she gets over-excited when there is someone to pay attention to her?

- Is she with adults most of the time?

- What kind of balance does she have between rest and activity?

These questions can lead you to ways of making her environment one that is stimulating without being too demanding. Remember that any attitude or behavior of yours that tends to make her feel guilty, ashamed, frustrated, inadequate, rejected, or anxious places her under pressure that often shows up in difficulty with the smooth flow of words. Many of these pressures can be reduced.

Monitor Overall Development.

Take a look at his development on the whole; physical skills and coordination, social skills, emotional and intellectual development. You may find that he is showing a special interest or rapid growth in any of these areas. If so, it may mean that his energy and attention will not be on speech skills for a time. His speech development is temporarily put aside so that he can concentrate on other areas.

Speech may appear to be less fluent than it was a few months before, or all his development may hit a general plateau. If this happens, try not to worry.

Development is not a continuous and steady process; growth often occurs in spurts. If this kind of plateau lasts too long, naturally you should look for reasons. You may then want to consult professional help. But if you see that he is intensely interested in learning to ride a tricycle, don't worry if his speech is set aside for awhile.

Consider Other Influences.

We have said that painful, traumatic incidents do not usually cause stuttering, but family tragedies naturally upset any child. In spite of your efforts to protect her, events such as illness, emotional conflict, moving, or accidents are sure to happen. They may be accompanied by a greater number of hesitations and repetitions in your child's speech.

If so, accept this as normal; don't add to her concern by reacting to her stuttering. If family conflicts continue, she may have more disfluencies. To counteract this, pay special attention to your loving relationship with her. If you take extra time and effort at these difficult times, your child's speech will probably return to its usual level of fluency.

Reduce Interruptions.

It is easy to interrupt someone who has many hesitancies in his speech; and if your child is showing signs of stuttering, this is to be avoided. You should not attempt to completely eliminate interruptions, but work hard to reduce them. Be alert for times when what he is saying is of special importance to him and try to avoid any interruptions then.

Look for other things that make it difficult for him to be as fluent as he can. Does he have more trouble talking and doing something else at the same time? Encourage him to stop the other activity when he wants to speak. If he is hurt while playing or over-excited for some reason, don't ask for explanations until he has calmed down. With some effort, you will be able to find many situations throughout the day when a little change in the way you do things will make it easier for him to speak more fluently.

Suggestion 5: Manage Your Child's Behavior

Self-doubts and feelings of failure arise when you make demands on your child to measure up to some ideal image. Are you demanding a level of perfection that is too high? Speech difficulties often arise during such episodes and may become conditioned to these feelings.

Have Appropriate Expectations for Behavior.

We sometimes expect our children to do or say certain things because it is socially correct to do so. If you expect your child to always be at his best, you are expecting too much.

Have tolerance for his age and abilities. Learning the right way to act or the right things to say takes time. He will learn by your own example, and he'll especially want to be like you if you praise him when he does well. Don't scold him or make him repeat his actions or words many times, thinking this will help him learn. After all, he is still a little child. If you are embarrassed by such behavior on his part, your expectations are too high.

Correct the Behavior, Not the Child.

Your child's misbehavior can be handled in such a way that other problems do not develop. Learning ways to manage her feelings and actions in positive ways is important.

If you make your child feel guilty and ashamed when she misbehaves, you are teaching her that she is bad. Instead, focus on teaching her that her *behavior* was wrong. You can do this by changing how you correct her. For example, instead of saying, "You are so naughty to your little sister!" try saying, "Pulling your sister's hair is naughty!" This points out her *behavior* caused a problem, rather than teaching her that *she* is the problem.

How do you handle her outbursts of anger? Obviously some controls are necessary. She needs to learn to manage this emotion effectively. If you treat it as something to be suppressed, the speech disfluencies that often occur at this time will become exaggerated in her mind. Any method you use to control her should avoid making her feel that she is bad because she has the emotion. Don't shame her in any way. You can calmly discuss her behavior afterward and explain there are many ways to cope with her feelings. This will help emphasize the difference between **having** a feeling and what one **does** with it.

Listen to your own language when you are angry with your child. Regardless of how you handle an immediate crisis, how do you follow up?

She needs explanations in order to know what you wanted to teach her when you were angry. You should help her to understand that you felt a need to release your own feelings. One way or another, she needs an explanation. Don't expect her to change her behaviors at once—she needs time and experience—but encourage improvement.

Be Consistent with Discipline.

There are some general guidelines to follow that will affect your child's feelings toward himself and others. Anything that gives him a feeling of being a failure may make him hesitate in speaking. At the same time, you need to teach him to behave appropriately and to act in ways that are reasonably comfortable for you and the rest of the family. The way in which you do this will have a direct influence on his feelings about himself.

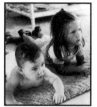

The way you use speech to punish or reward him is also important. Words and expressions can be as strong and as painful as a spanking. Using words this way may make him easy to control, but the cost is too high.

When you yell or punish him in other ways, how does he react? Does he freeze or look as if he is terribly afraid? Or do you completely miss his reaction because you are so angry? In either case, you are using your emotion as a club to force him to behave. This approach may work for a time but only at the sacrifice of his security. Another emotional club some parents use is: "If you love me and want me to love you, you must always do what I want you to do." Remember to focus on his behavior and let him know that his behavior is unacceptable, but that you know he can change how he behaves and you love him no matter what.

Examine all your methods of discipline: rewards and punishments. To what degree do they represent an objective and loving attitude on your part? Try to avoid methods that are too emotional, too prolonged, or too cold and stern. Use your own good judgment. You don't want to be erratic or random about your disciplining, nor do you want to be too rigid.

Control Excitement.

Special holidays, upcoming vacations, or starting preschool are exciting times, but they can be too stimulating for a young child. Parents often tell us that their child was fluent all summer but began to have trouble just before school started.

If you notice less fluency during these times, you should try to reduce the intensity of the situation. Sometimes the source of trouble is a high peak of excitement that lasts over too long a period of time. Christmas Day can cause a combination of high excitement plus frus-

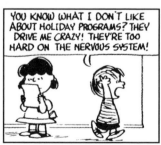

tration. One family handled this problem by taking most of the day to open presents. As each child opened a present, she would have time to play with the toy, try on her new clothes, or have part of a new book read to her. In this way, excitement was kept at a more pleasurable level. The children were not frustrated by too much too fast. The same can be done for birthdays.

When you are worried about your child, it shows. You may begin to treat him differently, lose patience more easily, or do other things that are different from how you normally interact with him. He is very sensitive to your own stress and concerns, so the best way to help him is to make sure you take care of yourself first.

If you are worried about your child's stuttering, getting information about it can help you feel better. You are on your way just by reading this book. Take action by following the suggestions in this book. This will help you feel less worried, because you are **doing** something for him rather than just thinking and worrying about his problem.

Monitor Brothers and Sisters.

If your child has brothers or sisters, you are well aware of how much they can help or hinder her development. They stimulate her to talk—and then they won't give her a chance to do it. Like baby birds in a nest, your children all compete for your attention in their own individual ways, and the one who speaks the quickest and loudest often succeeds in getting it.

The child with a tendency to stutter often needs to have controls put on the rest of the family to make sure she has a fair opportunity to speak. If she is inclined to be more withdrawn and hesitant than the others, she needs support from you more often. You can encourage her to talk by saying to brothers or sisters, "I wonder what your sister thinks about this?" then looking at her so that she knows it's her turn. If brothers or sisters interrupt, stop them and let them know it's not their turn right now and that they can have a turn when she is finished speaking.

This does not mean that she should always be allowed to talk, nor should you have rigid rules that the other children never interrupt her. Be sensible. All children need to learn to take turns in conversation. If you are overprotective of your child because of her stuttering, she will begin to do more of whatever it is that gives her the advantage over others. Be flexible in determining when you need to protect her right to talk and when she needs to give others a turn to talk themselves.

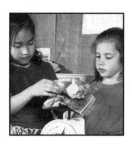

When she has a crisis of any kind, she should get more attention, just as each of the other children should, but the crisis must be real and not made-up. When in doubt, give her the attention.

Although they communicate in different ways, all of your children should have a chance to be heard. These differences are desirable; they give your children distinct personalities.

This attitude towards differences should carry over to those outside the family as well. Avoid using differences in personal characteristics to demean or downgrade anyone. If your child sees that you don't like people who look different or are disabled, in effect you are telling your child that differences are bad. He will then assume his own difference, such as difficulty in speaking, is also bad.

Suggestion 6: Use Common Sense

We have provided some general guidelines and a few specific suggestions for constructive ways of relating to your child. We hope you will be reasonable, thoughtful, and consistent in what you do, but we do not want to impose rigid patterns.

One mother was advised to establish a routine to give her son a sense of security. She set up such a tight schedule from 7 a.m. through 8 p.m. that every half hour had exactly the same activity every day. Needless to say, this routine created additional problems. A reasonable schedule and more relaxation on the part of the mother resulted in much improved fluency.

Avoid extremes. Pay attention to the effects of whatever you do and be ready to make adjustments in your actions and expectations when you see the need.

Part V

when stuttering seems more severe

Your child may worry you because for some reason or another, he seems to be much less fluent than you think he should be. Whether he is stuttering or not, you can be substantially reassured by the suggestions we have already provided. However, it may already be apparent to you and to the speech pathologist that your child is much more disfluent than he is expected to be at his age. In this case you will need to pay special attention to certain additional procedures. The suggestions that follow are ways of encouraging better fluency and preventing the development of severe stuttering. If you need more specifics for your unique situation, the speech pathologist can help you.

Reduce Time Pressure

Time pressure may adversely affect anyone's speech but particularly that of a young child. Although time pressures come in various forms, there are two types you should be aware of: 1) communicative and 2) lifestyle.

Communicative Time Pressure.

One good example of communicative time pressure is when a listener reacts - either with words or with body language - to a child's disfluencies by saying "slow down," "take your time," "relax." Or when a listener reacts in just the opposite way: "hurry up and spit it out," "I don't have all day...". Some listeners will tell the child to "slow down" one minute and then to "speed up, I don't have all day" the next!

Whichever way the adult listener reacts, the child may get the message that "I'd better try to speak as slowly (or as fast) as they want me to." Experience indicates that children are given these sorts of instructions, they have trouble maintaining normally fluent speech.

Instead of trying to **tell** your child to slow down or speed up, **show** her an appropriate rate of speech. In

...use a slower rate of speech...

order to do this you will need to examine and then possibly change some of **your own** speaking behaviors, at least when speaking with your child.

If you think that she is "talking too fast," study and listen to your own rate of speech when talking with her. We have heard parents tell their child to "slow down" while speaking themselves at a breakneck speed! We encourage you to spend some time listening to the speaking rate of slower adult talkers, a good example of which is Fred Rogers of Mister Rogers' Neighborhood. This will give you an idea about the way you can begin to slow down your own speech.

Try to spend five minutes each day using this slower rate of speech with your child. Lengthening the pauses **between** your words, phrases, and sentences should help you slow yourself down. Remember, the **way** you speak says more to your child than all of your verbal instructions to "slow down," "relax," or "speed up."

Adult listeners can also add to time pressure by finishing a child's sentences for him, jumping in the split second he is done, or beginning to talk before he even finishes his sentence. *Wait your child out—let him finish his sentence—and delay your own response by a second or two.*

As you begin to (1) speak more slowly in his presence (2) allow him to complete his sentence as well as delay by a second or so your own reply, you will be **showing** rather than telling your child how to talk in a way that will promote smoother, more fluent speech. Remember, making these changes in your speech, even for five minutes a day, will not be easy! You will probably find yourself having more success in slightly delaying your responses, not finishing sentences for him, and not talking before he finishes speaking than you will trying to slow down your own rate of speech.

Any and all changes you make towards a slower less rushed way of speaking will be helpful to your youngster. We know that this won't be easy but just do the best you can.

Lifestyle Time Pressure

A good example of the second kind of time pressure, lifestyle, is when parents set rigid, inflexible, arbitrary schedules for the times when the child must get up, eat breakfast, lunch, and dinner, take out the trash, go to bed, and so on. More often than not, the parent does this in an attempt to put some order into the chaos and confusion that often exists in a busy household. Whatever the reason, when parents require small children to run their lives in strict agreement with the clock on the wall, they often find themselves defeated and frustrated. Besides, it takes so much energy to enforce these time schedules and rules.

Another example of lifestyle time pressure is when families are constantly going from one activity to the next with few or no breaks in between. Not leaving enough time to get ready for preschool or daycare in the morning so that your child has to rush to get out the door on time can place time pressure on your child.

Parents are encouraged to examine their own possibly time-urgent lifestyle—**everything must be done on time**—and look for small ways in which they can change. Remember this: you have taken a lifetime to develop habits like having everything happen exactly on the dot, doing everything yourself so it will be done quickly, or not leaving enough time between events so that you're constantly rushing. You can't expect yourself to change such habits overnight. However, when you see the positive effect that reducing a time urgent, time scheduled existence has on your child and on yourself, we are sure that you will take the time to do everything in a little less rushed way!

Accept the Disfluencies

You probably have difficulty accepting your child's hesitant speech because you are afraid that she will develop lifelong stuttering. Even if you try to react unemotionally, the underlying feelings and attitudes will show through and have an effect on your child. To combat this, you will need to develop an understanding of all kinds of speech disfluencies, many of which are very common in everyday speech.

Study Speech Differences

Listen to the speech of other children and adults now and then, particularly when they are not talking to you. Count the disfluencies: any stoppage in the flow of words such as repetitions, back-tracking, pauses or insertions of extraneous noises. Become aware of how much disfluency appears in normal speech. Notice, too, how many different types of disfluency there are. Pauses are often used for emphasis, grammatical clarity, or for thinking and are perfectly normal interruptions. If you listen to your own breaks in fluency, you will find yourself becoming very sensitive to them. You will be impressed by how often disfluencies occur as part of everyone's general flow of speech.

Your child probably has more of these breaks in fluency than you do. You should note the variation and frequency of these. There will even be times when your child will be perfectly fluent.

This should reassure you because it shows you that he really does know how to talk and that with continued practice he can improve, although he cannot and will not be perfect all the time— nor should he be. As a result, you will begin to consider disfluencies in a different perspective.

Increase Your Tolerance for Disfluencies

The same amount of disfluency that causes one listener to become nervous may not even be noticed by another. If you find that your child's disfluencies continue to disturb you, you should try to increase your tolerance of them.

Asking yourself the following questions should lead you to a greater acceptance.

- Why are you irritated or upset when your child takes longer to say something than you think she should?
- Are you expecting a level of fluency she cannot meet?
- Why do you expect her to speak more fluently than she does? Because other children her age are more fluent, or because your other children are?
- Is it important that she develop just as they do?
- Do you take the necessary time to hear what she has to say?

The best way to improve your relationship with her is to take the necessary time.

- Are you still worried that she may get worse?
- Do you feel that her hesitant speech is a sign of basic inferiority?
- Are you worried about what will happen to her when she goes to school?

All this may simply be adding to the trouble she is having.

Express Acceptance

Another important way you can help your child is by accepting his disfluencies. What does this mean? It means that you show your child, through your actions and through your words, that disfluencies do not change how you feel about him. How do you show that you accept someone else's behavior? Essentially you say to yourself, "I notice that he is doing this but it doesn't matter. My feelings toward him have not changed. Most of the time I don't even notice." You recognize that many skills develop at different rates in children but you don't react to these differences until they become extreme. Even then you usually don't do anything until a problem has lasted a long time.

One mother improved her acceptance of her child's broken speech by reviewing how she had reacted when he was learning to eat with a spoon. He fumbled and spilled food many times in a process that took several months and was still not perfect when she told us of this experience. She recalled that she had managed not to be upset by his awkwardness; she considered it normal and therefore was pleased when he succeeded. As the weeks passed, the spills became fewer even though some meals were still mild disasters. Gradually the child became quite proficient and she could accept his occasional difficulties without emotion. She realized that she should react to his speech development in the same way.

We realize how difficult it may be for you to carry out these instructions if your child is stuttering severely. It may help you to remember that he is doing the best he can. So are you. When you react emotionally, you make him struggle harder to stop, avoid, or conceal his stuttering and this makes it worse. Don't make his problem more complex than it already is.

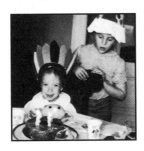

Describe the Behavior Rather Than Label It

We also recognize that this distinction between normal disfluencies and stuttering or abnormal disfluencies is not always made by the public in general. People often say, "I stutter once in awhile myself," or "Everyone stutters," when they are actually referring to normal disfluencies.

Perhaps you or others in the family have already labeled your child's speech stuttering or called him a stutterer. In this case, you should not make a desperate and sudden effort never to mention them for the reasons given above. Use descriptive terms instead of a label. Explain that he is repeating certain words, sounds, or syllables or that he is hesitating, interrupting his speech, stopping, pausing, or inserting extra sounds. Of course any word or expression can take on a negative connotation if used with vocal inflections or facial expressions that designate them as undesirable. The word disfluency, which we have used throughout this book, is intended to be a neutral term but could well become as negative as the label stuttering if used in the wrong way.

If your child struggles intensely and often with his disfluencies and shows anxiety and fear, you will need to do more than simply accept his speech. You should continue to use as many descriptive terms as possible when discussing stuttering with him. If you notice tense muscles, eye blinks, reluctance to attempt words, mouth postures with no sounds coming out or similar behaviors, you could tell him that he struggles or works too hard. At the same time, you should not make special efforts to conceal the label from him if everyone else is thinking of his speech as stuttering. **Complete avoidance of the word in these circumstances makes him more anxious, not less. It isn't the words which are bad but the way in which they are used.**

One term should be avoided. Try not to see him as "a stutterer." There is a subtle but critical difference between "he is a stutterer," and "He stutters." The former sets him apart as a separate person; the latter says he is **doing** something just as he does a lot of things.

Reduce Your Anxiety

We are aware of your difficulty in listening to your child stutter and of your natural anxiety about him. One mother who brought her child to the speech clinic expressed how worn out and overwhelmed she felt as her child struggled with his speech. Difficult as it may seem, you can do something about your own anxiety.

Remember that most children who stutter do not continue to do so after childhood. Your understanding, help, and support when the problem is still in its early stages greatly increases the probability that your child will achieve normal fluency.

Your ability to look at stuttering objectively and to understand what he is doing—and we can all modify or change the way we do things—should help you reduce your anxiety. Your efforts to determine its severity and consistency give you something positive to work on. Be conscious of your increasing ability to observe his stuttering calmly and to refrain from becoming tense or alarmed when he suddenly stutters.

Concentrate on what is happening now and not on what might happen in years to come. Determine how much fluency he has. If you count his words for a period of time, noting the difficulties, you will find that an overwhelming percentage of the words are perfectly normal—not all of them perfectly fluent, but certainly acceptable for his age. You have ample evidence here that he does know how to talk.

When the factors which increase or aggravate his intermittent stuttering are reduced, he will be freer to talk without undue interruptions. In the meantime, you and he have a problem that is best worked out if you are not too anxious.

React Appropriately to Stuttering

Stuttering could become so disturbing to your child and so distracting that a total lack of reaction on your part would be inappropriate. In this case, you should show him that you recognize what he did without showing any hint of surprise, criticism or pity.

Nor should you suggest that he do something about it. You might say, "That word is really tricky, isn't it," or "You worked hard on that word," or "Some words are hard to say, aren't they." These should be presented as statements of fact. Other times, just try a smile with a look and word that says, "Sometimes words just don't come out easily."

Occasionally his combinations of sounds and timing will be funny; laugh with him and go on with the conversation. You can even display mild sympathy for him. The vocal inflection and timing of these reactions are vital. In the speech clinic we often observe parents who have learned to handle this problem beautifully. One mother changed her horror of stuttering into an attitude of admiration for her son who managed to communicate well in spite of a severe problem, and this attitude was reflected in her voice.

We appreciate how difficult this is when you are worried or feeling sorry for your child as he struggles, but try not to add to his anxiety. You may need to work on your own feelings before you are able to react as we have outlined. We do not mean that you should stifle all feelings of sympathy for your child; just let this feeling come out in an attitude of constructive love that sees him as much more than "a stutterer." The problem is such a small part of what he is. It is just that – a problem which needs to be worked out like bed-wetting or nose-picking – which need to be managed sensibly.

Talk Openly about Stuttering

When your child goes to a speech pathologist, he may need to be told that because he is having trouble with words "getting stuck," you would like to have an expert listen to him and try to find ways to help. He may ask questions about his speech, such as "Why can't I talk?" "Why do I get stuck?" or even "What's the matter with me?" At other times, the look on your child's face when he is especially distressed may call for a positive response on your part. You may notice that he has the idea that stuttering should be hidden. **Your bringing it out into the open should help him**.

Answers to "Why do I stutter?" are the most difficult, but you can best satisfy him with short explanations. Here is an example of what you might tell him.

...talk openly about stuttering

All of us get tangled up or stuck at times. Some of us do it more than others. Little children are more likely to hesitate because they are still learning to talk. They also stumble more when walking and running. When they have trouble speaking, they sometimes try too hard to stop and this makes it worse.

By calling his attention to stumblings in your own speech when they occur, you can help him to understand that all of us sometimes have trouble talking. Any question about whether or not something is the matter with him should be answered by "no," and followed by a fuller description of what is happening when he stutters, such as, "you held onto that sound a little too long" or "that was a little bumpy." You can use these opportunities to reassure him that it is all right for him to get stuck if he feels he cannot speak any other way. The main idea is to be as descriptive as possible, to keep explanations simple and to avoid sounding mysterious or emotional.

Give Direct Advice at Times

After asking "Why?" your child may ask "How can I stop it?" The best suggestion is "Don't work so hard," or "Try to relax and loosen up the tightness." One parent demonstrated this idea by squeezing his fist and gradually relaxing it while letting a sound "leak out." You can show your child two ways of saying a word - the "hard" and the "easy" way to let a sound out. If he needs to repeat words or sounds he should try to do so in a relaxed way; it is the struggle that makes things worse. If he says he cannot talk in any other way, give him the time he needs. Above all, do not become irritated when he does not or cannot follow your advice.

Do not tell your child how **not** to stutter. Advice such as "Take a deep breath," or "Think of what you want to say before you speak," or "Slow down" will compound his problem in at least three ways:

1. It implies that if he did something right he would not stutter;
2. It makes him feel guilty because he cannot make the advice work; and
3. It often adds additional behaviors to his talking which distract him and his listeners and further impede the flow of speech.

Reduce Fears and Frustrations with Speech

One of the best ways to do this is to encourage your child to talk about her fears, anxieties, and frustrations. This means that you must be prepared to accept how she feels without criticism or disapproval, regardless of how irrational her feelings may seem to you. They are not signs of weakness or inadequacy; they show that she is human. One parent expressed his own fears, past and present, and was able to get the idea across to his daughter that everybody has fears—it's OK to have fears—and that we can all learn to reduce them.

Many of your child's fears may not be directly related to talking, but they can still have an overall effect on her by making her more hesitant and withdrawn. Bringing her fears out in the open and reassuring your child that you accept her and her fears can greatly reduce their importance.

Encourage Independence

Avoid increasing your child's fears by overprotection. Don't do everything for him or arrange his life in such a way that he doesn't need to talk. If he will talk on the telephone, encourage it. Overprotection will eventually add to his fears of talking and stuttering.

Deal with Fears in Small Steps

There are additional ways to deal with your child's fears. Many parents allow their child to have a dim night-light to offset fear of the dark. Try approaching that which causes her fear in steps, and stop temporarily when she shows any fear. Then move towards the source of fear when she is ready. Never force her; take the necessary time.

One child would run from the room whenever visitors came to the home. His mother helped him by waiting until the guests were seated and talking, then she called the child to the door to get something from her; the first time it was a piece of cake she was serving. In later visits, the child was able to sit quietly in her lap for part of the visit and to say "goodbye" when he left. The barriers were thus gradually overcome.

Teach Your Child to Cope with Frustration

If your child encounters periods of very severe blocking and stuttering, he will probably build up a great deal of frustration. Many parents describe various ways of coping effectively with this. One encouraged her son to hit an inflated Bobo the Clown as hard as he could until he felt better. Another talked to his son in private and allowed the child to say what he wanted without any disapproval, only reassurance that he understood the child's feelings. Outdoor exercise is also helpful in reducing tension as are any activities where expression is nonverbal.

A Parting Word

We have outlined many things for you to do in order to ensure your child the best chance of developing normal fluency. As you carry out our suggestions, try to go a little further. Look for ways to give more of yourself to your child, by spending more time, by playing and talking with your child, and in showing interest in his interests.

Do these things not just because your child stutters, but for the mutual pleasure of being together. Do not seek or expect appreciation. You are not doing a favor that deserves special thanks, but instead just being a more warm and responsive parent.

You may also want to ask the speech pathologist for methods appropriate to your specific situation. If you create your own, they will probably work better than ours. Just try to keep in mind the general principles we have described for a constructive and positive relationship with your child.

Obtaining Reimbursement for Stuttering Treatment

Approximately three million children and adults in the U.S. stutter. This guide provides suggestions and resources for obtaining payment for the treatment of stuttering.

1. Will my health plan cover stuttering treatment?

Before contacting your health plan, review your policy for coverage looking for such terms as "speech therapy," "speech-language pathology," "physical therapy and other rehabilitation services," or "other medically necessary services or therapies." A phone call to the health plan can confirm your interpretation of coverage. Document the name of the person with whom you speak as well as dates and times.

Provide the health plan with information about the neurological basis of stuttering, which states:

"Researchers who studied adults with persistent stuttering found that these individuals had anatomical irregularities in the areas of the brain that control language and speech." *Neurology* (July 24, 2001)

When speaking with the health plan representative, it may be helpful to provide the **diagnostic code** for stuttering (typically **307.0**) and the **treatment codes** for stuttering: **92506** for speech evaluation, **92507** for **individual** speech treatment, and **92508** for **group** speech treatment.

Be sure to get the name of the health plan representative with whom you talked and ask for confirmation of coverage in writing. Specifics of coverage (e.g., any limit on the number of sessions, co-payments, deductible amounts, etc.) should also be provided in writing. The health plan should provide this written notification within 30 to 60 days.

If treatment for stuttering is not covered by your policy, ask the health plan to explain the reasons for the denial in writing. This information can be helpful in appealing the original determination.

Keep copies of all correspondence and detailed records of all verbal communication.

2. Does the health plan require a physician referral before payment for the treatment of stuttering?

Some insurers do require this pre-approval. Your policy booklet or your insurance representative should be able to tell you if your policy requires a referral from your primary physician prior to beginning treatment for stuttering. Pre-approval may be a form that your primary physician completes and submits to the health plan. Pre-approval may also require a letter of referral, which is submitted along with your insurance form to the health plan.

If a letter is required for pre-approval of treatment for stuttering, it should contain the following information:

_____ is a patient of mine with neuro-oral-muscular discoordination resulting in stuttering, which interferes with his/her oral communication. In order to treat this disorder, it is medically necessary that my patient receive specialized, comprehensive speech treatment from _____.

Typically, the health plan also requires a form from the speech-language pathologist, which includes the diagnostic and treatment codes for stuttering, projected treatment dates or number of treatment sessions anticipated, as well as associated fees. The health plan is required to notify you within 30 to 60 days as to the status of approval.

3. How do I submit a claim?

Speech treatment for stuttering is usually conducted in one of two ways: weekly sessions or intensive, short-term treatment programs.

A. Weekly Sessions

If speech treatment is provided once or twice a week, claims can be submitted in a number of ways: at the completion of each session, after a block of sessions, or filed with a projected number of sessions. If more sessions are needed than originally anticipated, a progress report is submitted to the health plan with a request for coverage for additional sessions. The speech-language pathologist can assist you in determining the best way to submit your claim, or may submit the claim for you.

B. Intensive Short-Term Treatment

If treatment is provided through an intensive short-term treatment program, the claim must be submitted at the completion of the program. Intensive short-term treatment programs are typically conducted over a 2–4 week period.

Once the treatment program is completed, the speech-language pathologist will supply the appropriate diagnostic and treatment codes and either you or the clinician will submit this information, along with your insurance form, to the health plan.

Regardless of the type of treatment program recom-mended—weekly or intensive, short-term—you should call the health plan a week after mailing the claim to make certain it has been received.

4. What can I do if my claim is denied?

If your claim is denied, request the reasons for denial **in writing**. You have the right to appeal the denial. Remember, persistence often pays off.

First, write a letter stating your intention to appeal the denial. The health plan may request additional information about the treatment and/or they may ask for an objective measurement of progress. They may cite as a reason for denial that treatment is "educational in nature" or that treatment is not "medically necessary". Your appeal must address the specific reasons for denial.

An appeal letter typically includes a description of the disorder and its medical nature. A copy of the physician's referral letter (if pre-approval was needed) should be included. It may be helpful to quote those sections of the policy booklet that describe the coverage for speech-language pathology treatment, if it helps your case. Then you will need to describe how the treatment meets the policy criteria.

In any correspondence with the health plan:

- Use terms that are **medically oriented** (e.g., evaluation, diagnosis, condition) rather than behavioral or learning theory terminology (e.g., test, examination, teach).
- Do not include the time of onset of stuttering, unless specifically requested.
- Include estimated length of treatment if known.
- Indicate that treatment is provided by an ASHA certified, and licensed where applicable, speech-language pathologist and include the clinician's ASHA membership number and state license number.

- Demonstrate significant practical improvement using objective, measurable terms.
- Document improvement by indicating how the patient has applied progress in treatment to real life situations (may be referred to as functional outcomes).

Your speech-language pathologist can help you with this appeal. Sample appeal letters are also available through the American Speech-Hearing-Language Association (ASHA).

Once the health plan receives the information, they must respond within a time period of 30 to 60 days depending upon the state. **Follow up and persistence can lead to success!**

5. What action can I take if my appeal is denied?

If you feel that your appeal has been unfairly denied or that your case was handled unprofessionally or inappropriately, there is action that can be taken.

- Contact your state insurance commissioner to determine if there are any other instances in which claims have been unfairly denied and/or file a complaint. Contact information for your insurance commissioner can be found by contacting the Publications Department of the National Association of Insurance Commissioners by phone (816-783-8300), by fax (816-460-7593), or by e-mail (www.naic.org).
- Contact the American Speech-Language-Hearing Association by phone (1-800-498-2071) or by e-mail (www.asha.org) or your state speech-language-hearing association. Your speech-language pathologist can provide you with contact information for your state speech-language-hearing association.
- Contact the Stuttering Foundation of America by phone 1-800-992-9392, visit us at www.stutteringhelp.org, or e-mail us at info@stutteringhelp.org.
- Recommend to your employer or union that coverage for speech-language treatment should be included in your health benefits plan.
- Consider filing a claim in small claims court or state court if all other efforts fail.

6. Are there any other ways to pay for treatment?

There are other ways to pay for treatment if you are having difficulty financing yourself. Here are some alternatives:

- Most states have an agency that helps handicapped or disabled individuals. The names vary from state to state but are usually called Departments of Vocational Rehabilitation. You can find your state's department by calling information at your sate capitol. Contact the agency to see if you qualify. Most states require a minimum age of 18 for vocational rehabilitation services.
- You can request financial help from your local civic organizations like the Elks Club, Lions, Rotary, SERTOMA, Etc.

Reference this material as follows: American Speech-Language-Hearing Association Special Interest Division 4, Fluency and Fluency Disorders and Stuttering Foundation of America (1998; Revised 2002). *Obtaining reimbursement for stuttering treatment.* Rockville MD: Author.

Finding Professional Help

The Stuttering Foundation at 1-800-992-9392 and www.stutteringhelp.org (www.tartamudez.org in Spanish) will provide you with the names of speech-language pathologists who specialize in stuttering. In addition, agencies that may provide speech testing and therapy include your local school district (contact your local elementary school for more information), a hospital clinic (look under "Outpatient Services" or "Speech Therapy"), or a speech and hearing clinic at a nearby university.

No matter whom you choose, be sure to ask:

- Have you / has the therapist who will see my child had a lot of experience working with those who stutter?
- Are you / is this therapist experienced in working with children?
- Do you / does the therapist have certification from the American Speech-Language-Hearing Association (CCC-SLP)?